RAPID WEIGHT GAIN SMOOTHIES

STRENGTH TRAINING BODYBUILDING HIGH PROTEIN SHAKES FOR FAST MUSCLE MASS BUILDING

Steve R. Gansneder

ISBN-13:978-1973919698

ISBN-10:1973919699

CONTENTS

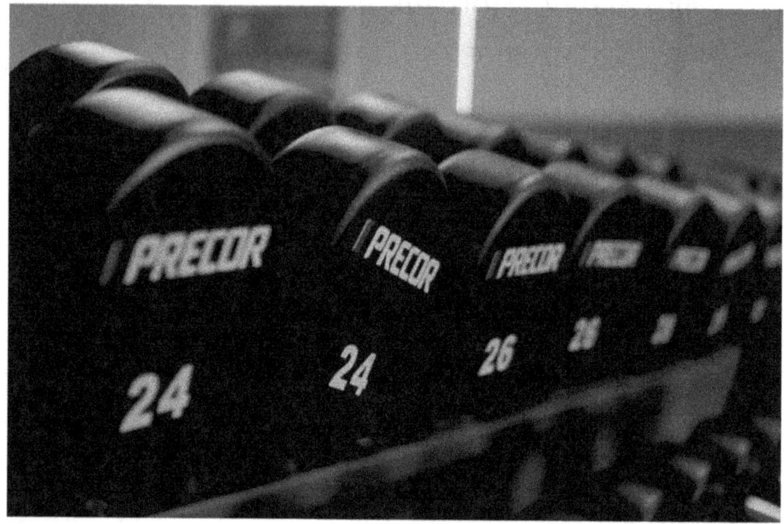

The art of gaining weight is based upon consuming more calories and building lean muscle.

In order to gain one pound, a total of 3,500 additional calories are required. It's difficult to consume 3,500 healthy calories from three meals and two snacks a day. For this reason, when a high protein, high calorie smoothie is incorporated into the daily regime it results in weight gain.

Energy input comes in the form of proteins, carbohydrates and lipids, basically from the foods we consume. Proteins provide 4 kcal of energy per gram, carbohydrates provide 4kcal/gram, and lipids provide 9 kcal/gram. Energy output is conducted by the basal metabolic rate, the thermal effect of food (how much energy is used to digest food), thermogenesis (non voluntary physical activity, i.e. leg bouncing, fidgeting) and physical exercise. When energy input and output are balanced, weight is maintained. When energy input is greater than output, weight gain results. When energy output is greater than input, weight loss results.

The body's basal metabolic rate is basically the rate of energy that is required to be alive, and it changes with the activity level. Factors that increase the basal metabolic rate are: % of lean body mass (muscle burns more calories than fat), gender (men have higher BMI), body surface per body volume (tall/short), body temperature, thyroid hormones (if elevated, BMR lowers), stress, pregnancy, caffeine and tobacco. When attempting to gain weight, it is important to gain and maintain lean muscle, usually in the form of resistance training. When lean body mass increases, so does the basal metabolic rate because lean tissue is more metabolically active than fat. The recipes in this book are based on the objectives of offering nutritionally dense foods and foods that provide the greatest energy input.

Safety Guidelines:

- Raw eggs are never safe in a recipe. Always an egg product that has been pasteurized.
- Make sure all vegetables and fruits are clean.
- Utensils, cutting boards, blenders should be clean..
- A sharp knife is a safe knife. Avoid using dull blades.
- Any remaining ingredients should be used within 3 days to avoid food borne illness.

Adding Extra Calories, Protein and Fiber:

- Oats provide soluble and insoluble fiber. Add 1/2 - 1 cup to any recipe.
- Add nuts and seeds to the recipe to add heart-healthy oils. Consider flax, sunflower, pumpkin seeds, as well as walnuts, almonds or macadamia nuts.
- Nut butters add protein and thicken the smoothie. Sunflower butter, almond, cashew or peanut butter work great in smoothies.
- Try different flavors of powdered proteins.
- Ice cream is a great way to add protein to any of the smoothies.
- Yogurt or Kefir can be incorporated into any smoothie recipe to provide probiotics for healthy gut flora.

Lactose Intolerance

Those with lactose intolerance or casein allergies might consider substituting dairy products such as:

- Soy or almond milk
- Lactaid brand milk
- Dairy-free creamers
- Yogurt based on soy

Preparation

- Ensure veggies and fruits are clean.
- Combine ingredients in blender.
- Ice may be added as a thinning agent.

2000 CALORIE SMOOTHIE

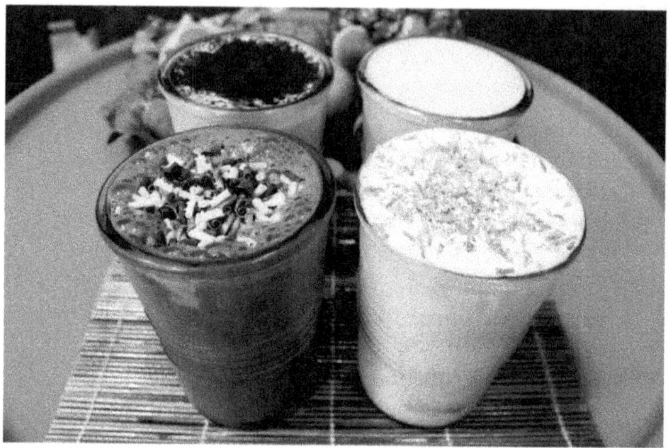

This 2000 calorie smoothie offers 93 grams of protein, which is tricky to consume on a daily basis through traditional meals. Imagine having to stop throughout the day and eat the ingredients individually! That in itself is a workout!

Delicious, quick and easy to make, this high calorie, high protein smoothie offers naturally occurring sugars from bananas and dairy, healthy oils (from the olive oil and peanut butter), and a good amount of fiber from the oats. Additionally, the bananas provide a great deal of potassium, which prevents muscle cramps. Whole milk and premium ice creams are recommended for this smoothie because they contain more fat.

It's ideal for those days when you're on the go, yet you still want to meet your daily target of protein to ensure minimal muscle loss.

Variety is the spice of life!

Vary flavored protein powders and dairy products: for example, use a strawberry flavored whey protein and combine with strawberry ice cream!

Vanilla protein with a touch of vanilla extract, and of course, vanilla ice cream!

Add smooth fruits like mango, avocado or papaya to enhance natural sweetness.

If you prefer not to have ice cream, substitute with two additional bananas.

Ingredients:

- 2 Cups Milk
- 2 Bananas
- 2 Scoops protein
- 1 Cup Ice Cream
- 2 Tbsp Olive Oil
- 1/2 Cup Oats
- 4 Tbsp Peanut Butter

Directions:

1. NOTE: Oats breakdown best if they are soaked in water for two minutes, or ground in a blender.
2. Combine in blender milk, bananas, ice cream and peanut butter.
3. Add oats and whey protein.Puree until blended.
4. While pureeing, drizzle in olive oil until all ingredients are fully combined.

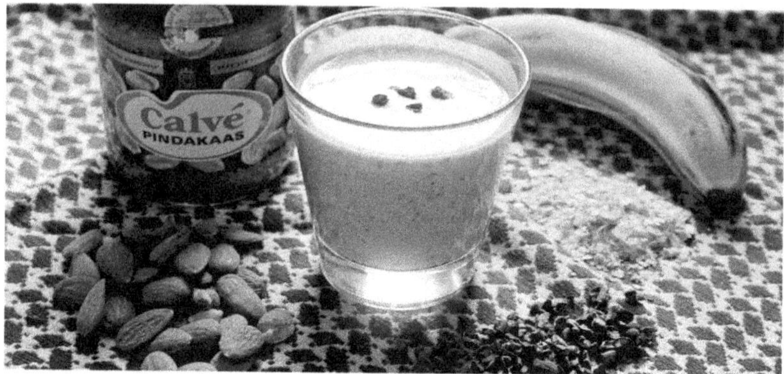

A classic favorite, this dairy-based shake offers 102 grams of protein and is delicious! Sweet, rich and thick, you won't believe this is actually good for you because it tastes fabulous!

This shake offers its nutritional and caloric counts primarily from dairy, protein powder, yogurt, almond butter. Fiber is gained through the oats and the Greek yogurt offers not only a silky smoothness, but is helpful to creating "a happy gut" by providing good bacteria to the digestive tract. Almond butter provides a bit of magnesium to diet. The objective of using coconut oil is to add medium length triglycerides to the diet. Medium chain triglycerides (MCT's) are a shorter chain s of fat that are absorbed intact and delivered directly to the liver, where they are stored and used as energy. When choosing a coconut oil, it is recommended you use a quality oil, as there are a great deal of coconut oils on the market that do not provide enough MCT's. The energy source of coconut oil should be listed on the label. You want at least 62% MCT's per serving.

Variety is the Spice of Life:

If you're looking for a sweeter shake, try these ideas!

Substitute granola for oats

Add a teaspoon of Agave nectar (Agave nectar vs. Honey: Agave nectar doesn't impact your glycemic index as much as honey)

Ingredients:

- 2 Cups Whole Milk
- 1.5 Cups Oatmeal

- 2 Scoops Protein Powder
- 1 Cup Greek Yogurt
- 2 Tbsp Almond Butter
- 1 Tbsp Coconut Oil
- 1 Banana

Directions:

NOTE: The oats breakdown best if they are soaked in water for two minutes, or ground in a blender.

- To the blender, add milk, banana, yogurt and almond butter. Puree until blended.
- Then add the whey powder and oats. Puree until blended.
- Add coconut oil and puree until all ingredients are fully combined.

PERFECT PALEO SHAKE

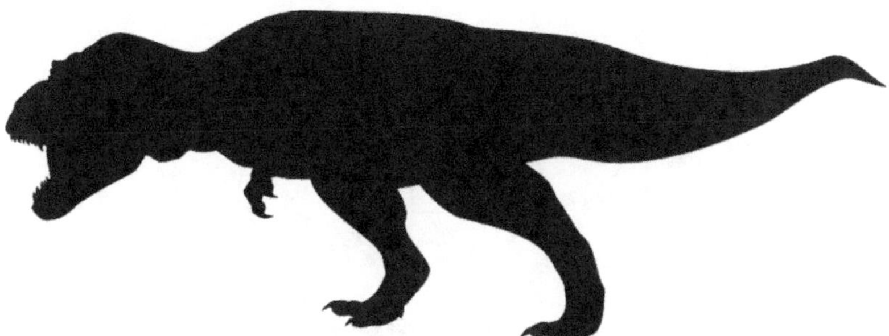

Perfect for the Paleo diet, this nutritious and tasty shake derives its caloric and nutritional values primarily from a banana, coconut and almond milk, nuts, and coconut oil, all of which provide 40 grams of protein. Do not be alarmed by the term "milk". The coconut and almonds are ground into liquids which produce oils from the nuts -- not milk. Bananas provide magnesium, potassium and vitamin C. Nuts and seeds are great sources of vitamins, minerals and Omega 3 oils.

Variety is the Spice of Life:

- Add any type of fruit to the recipe to sweeten --berries are ideal!
- Add seeds to the recipe for enhanced nutrition - sunflower, chia, pumpkin, or flax seeds

Nuts give the Paleo shake distinction- try using walnuts, which are super antioxidants, or raw almonds, which are also heart-healthy and packed with vitamin E. Other nuts to consider are brazil nuts, or pine nuts.

Ingredients:

- 1 Banana
- 2 tbsp Coconut Oil
- 1/2 Cup Mixed Nuts
- 1 Scoop Protein
- 1 Cup Coconut Milk
- 1 Cup Almond Milk

Directions:

1. Add all ingredients into blender and puree until blended thoroughly.

OPTION: add ice after all ingredients have been blended thoroughly for a cold shake

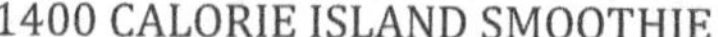

1400 CALORIE ISLAND SMOOTHIE

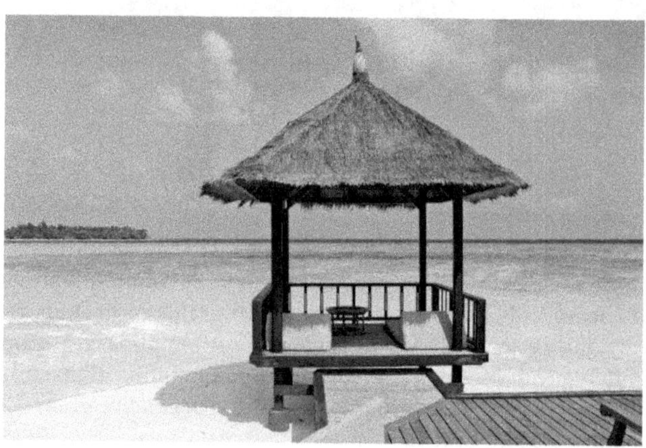

Dreaming of being on a beach, sipping a tropical drink? Then you've found your next vacation! This concoction is super refreshing and provides 52 grams of protein. Bananas and coconut are the major players in contributing to the caloric count. The fruits and their skins provide a whopping amount of vitamin C, as well as other essential vitamins and nutrients. So sit back, relax and enjoy island life!

Variety is the Spice of Life:

- Vary the flavor of protein - strawberry flavored protein works great with this recipe!
- Add fruit: Fresh pineapple is a natural for this recipe. It adds the enzyme Bromelain to the shake. Bromelain is an enzyme natural to pineapples. It has been shown to provide anti-inflammatory benefits, as well assist in breathing issues such as asthma.

Ingredients:

- 1 Banana
- 1 Cup Papaya
- 1 cup Mango
- 1 cup Coconut Milk
- 1 tbsp Shredded Coconut
- 1/4 cup Macadamia Nuts
- 2 Scoops Protein

Directions:

1. Chop nuts in blender to desired size.
2. Add milk, mango, papaya and banana. Puree until blended.
3. Add protein powder and coconut. Continue to blend to desired thickness. Add water, ice, or coconut water for a thinner smoothie.

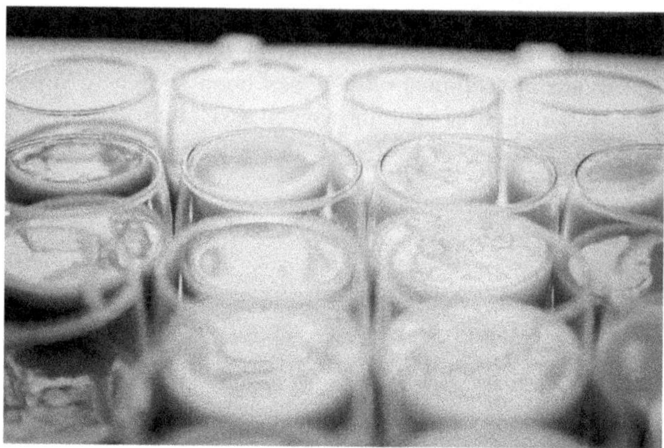

If you love the combination of bananas and walnuts, you'll love this smoothie that provides 46 grams of protein. The high caloric and nutrient content comes primarily from the butters. However, this smoothie offers a punch of iron through the fresh spinach. A bit of sweetness comes from the apple that offers thousands of nutritional benefits, and you'll get a good dose of Omega 3's from the avocado.

Variety is the Spice of Life:

Vary the greens: substitute spinach with kale

Want it sweeter? Add a little Agave Nectar

Ingredients:

- 1 Scoop Protein
- 1 Cup Walnuts
- 30g/1 Cup Spinach
- 1 Banana
- 1/2 Avocado
- 1/2 Apple
- 1 Tbsp Coconut Oil

Directions:

1. In a blender, pulse walnuts to desired size.
2. Combine remaining ingredients and puree until desired consistency.
3. Add ice or water to reduce consistency.

If you're looking for a weight gaining smoothie and following a Ketogenic diet, you've probably experienced disappointment in finding the right combination sans fruit. How can a smoothie be delicious if it has no fruit? This recipe meets your concerns and calms the taste buds by providing 54 grams of protein and offers   a low carbohydrate count. Calories from the butters, and sweetness from the heavy cream and almond milk make this a neato-keto smoothie!

Variety is the Spice of Life:

A good way to sweeten this smoothie is to use heavy cream instead of coconut cream

Use almond or sunflower butter in place of macadamia butter. Macadamia butter has 4 carbohydrates per 2 tablespoons versus almond butter and sunflower butter which have 6 and 4 carbohydrates, respectively.

Fruit - if you've just got to have a fruit in your smoothie, 1/2 cup of raspberries has 3 grams of carbohydrates, blackberries have 4 grams, strawberries have 6 grams, blueberries have 6 grams. These are the lowest fruit choices for a Ketogenic diet, and if you're on a strict Ketogenic diet, these fruits should be considered a "once in a while treat".

Ingredients:

- 1/2 Cup Almond Milk
- 1/2 Cup Heavy Cream
- 2 Tbsp Macadamia Butter
- 2 Tbsp Coconut Oil
- 2 Scoops Whey Protein

Directions:

1. In a blender, combine milk, cream, butter and oil. Puree until blended.
2. Add protein powder and blend until thoroughly incorporated.

Leafy greens provide a ton of nutrients, including protein, vitamins and minerals. Unfortunately, most of us don't eat enough greens. This tasty treat punches a whopping 66 grams of protein and meets your recommended daily allowance of vegetables. Which is better, kale or spinach? While both are remarkably nutrient dense, kale, is the most nutrient-dense green of the two. It provides a bit more protein and has four times the amount of vitamin C than spinach. Kale also provides more vitamin A (good for the eyes and skin) and vitamin K, which is important for bones and clotting. The banana and dates provide a bit of sweetness and dates are a great source of both soluble and insoluble fiber, which is great for digestion. For this recipe, you'll want to use pitted dates.

Variety is the Spice of Life:

Vary the Greens: other greens with impressive nutritional value are collards, celery, cucumber, dandelion, and romaine. You might enjoy adding some broccoli crowns, brussel sprouts or asparagus.

Sweeten: add an apple or a bit of Agave nectar

Ingredients:

- 1/2 Cup Dates
- 3 Bananas
- 1 Cup Kale
- 1 Cup Spinach
- 1/2 Cup Blueberries
- 1 Tbsp Olive Oil
- 1 Cup Milk
- 2 Scoops Protein

Directions:

1. Combine milk and all ingredients except oil and protein powder. Puree till blended thoroughly.
2. Add the protein powder. Puree.
3. Continue to blend smoothie while drizzling in oil.

This sweetie provides approximately half of the recommended daily allowances of iron, vitamin C and antioxidants, as well has a healthy dose of fiber from the oats. In all, it contains 66 grams of protein and can be made in an instant! The berries also provide antioxidants which are necessary for removing free radicals in the body. This recipe calls for Creatine Powder which can be found at most health food stores. Creatine is a natural compound made by the body to provide energy to cells. This energy is called adenosine triphosphate, or ATP. It's made in the liver and stored in the brain, muscles, testes and heart.

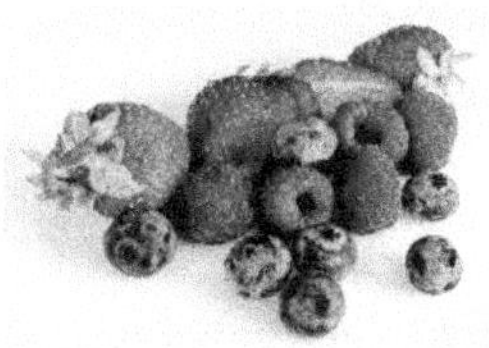

Creatine circulates throughout our bodies, taking care of us at the cellular level. Once we have enough ATP, or cellular energy, the remainder of creatine is converted to creatinine, and is excreted through the kidneys.

Variety is the Spice of Life:

Vary the flavor of protein powder

Sweeten with a tad of Agave nectar

Add greens - kale, spinach

Ingredients:

- 1 cup oats
- 1 cup whole milk
- 1/2 cup raspberries
- 1/2 cup blueberries
- 2 bananas
- 1 Peach
- 2 scoops of protein powder
- 1 scoop of Creatine powder

Directions:

1. Combine and puree oats to the desired consistency.
2. You can also soak the oats in water for a few minutes to soften them.
3. Blend the oats into a powder.
4. Remove the peach pit. (You can peel the peach or not. Soft fruit skins contain many nutrients.)
5. Add remaining ingredients and puree to desired consistency.

You'll want to keep these three simple ingredients tucked away in the kitchen as they are a fabulous base for just about any vegan smoothie and, they provide 14 grams of protein. Bananas, dates and coconut water-that's it!!! This raw and vegan combination provides a semi-sweet starting point so use your imagination and go for it! Pitted dates are recommended for this recipe and they provide a nice punch of soluble and insoluble fiber. Coconut water is one of the most hydrating waters and in its virgin state, it doesn't taste like coconuts! You can, however, buy coconut-flavored coconut water, or even lemon-lime flavored coconut water.

Variety is the Spice of Life:

Spice it up: add cinnamon, nutmeg

Sweeten: add any fresh fruit - papaya, mango, passion fruit, berries

Chill it: add ice to blender

Ingredients:

- 5 Bananas
- 1 Cup Dates
- 2 Cups Coconut Water

Directions:

1. Combine all three ingredients and blend to desired consistency. Note: if the dates aren't breaking down as you'd like, add a bit of water and puree them first. Then add the other two ingredients.

The basic premise behind this recipe is to "eat all your colors". This colorful smoothie provides 63 grams of protein, as well an assortment of vitamins, nutrients and minerals, including vitamins A, C and E, calcium, iron, fiber and potassium. If you prefer spinach to kale, remember spinach shrinks more than kale during processing, so buy double the amount. Pitted dates are recommended.

Variety is the Spice of Life:

Vary greens: substitute spinach for kale

Add color: red raspberries, blueberries, blackberries, apricot, orange, peach, nectarine or plums

Ingredients:

- 3 Bananas
- 1 Cup Blueberries
- 1 Cup Raspberries
- 1 Cup Strawberries
- 1 Tbsp Almond Butter
- 1/4 Cup Dates
- 1 Cup Kale
- 1 Tbsp Olive Oil
- 2 Scoops Protein

Directions:

1. Combine berries in blender and puree to desired consistency.
2. Add dates and puree.
3. Add remaining ingredients and continue to blend to desired consistency.

NUTTY BANANA SMOOTHIE

The most purchased fruit in the world, bananas are creamy, filling and always satisfying. This nutty banana smoothie provides a host of healthy benefits. Magnesium, potassium, calcium and vitamins come from the bananas and the nuts provide a healthy dose of Omega 3's and carbohydrates.

Ingredients:

- 2 Large Bananas
- 4-5 Walnuts and 4-5 Cashews
- ½ Cup Milk
- ½ Cup Yogurt
- 1 Scoop of Whey Protein Powder
- 3-4 Ice Cubes

Directions:

- Combine ice, banana, milk, yogurt to blender and puree to desired consistency.
- Add ice to combination and puree.
- Add nuts and whey powder. Combine to desired consistency.
- Add banana and puree until smooth.

PBS SMOOTHIE

This smoothie is a refreshing spin on the PBJ (peanut, butter, jelly) we ate as kids. The nut butter provides protein and the strawberry provides vitamins and antioxidants. This is a very simple recipe and kids love it when made with strawberry flavored protein powder.

Ingredients:

- 1 Cup Strawberry
- 2 Tablespoon of Peanut butter
- ½ Cup of Milk
- 1 Scoop of Whey Protein Powder
- 3-4 Ice Cubes

Directions:

1. Combine all ingredients, except powder. Puree until smooth.
2. Add protein powder. (Note: Strawberry flavored protein powder is recommended).

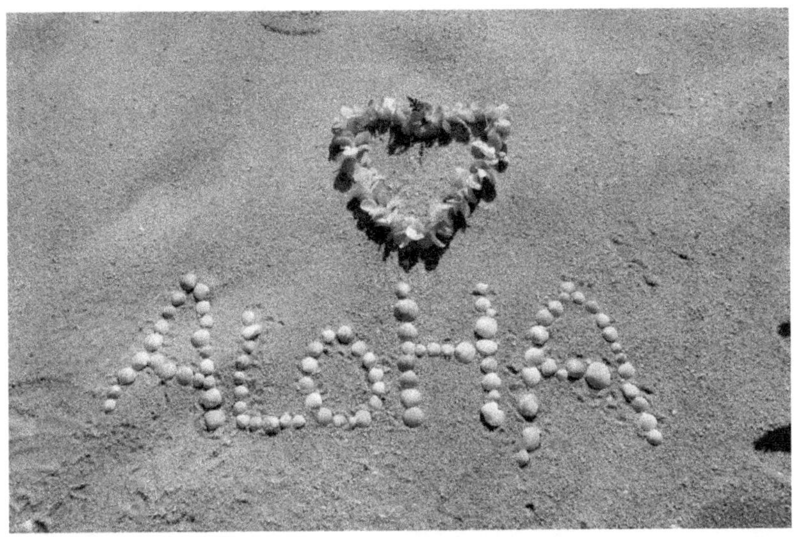

This smoothie reminds one of relaxing on the island of Maui because pineapple is the key ingredient! It is important to use fresh pineapple because the nutritional properties of canned versus fresh are quite different. Canned pineapple is often packed in a syrup, which contains added sugars. Fresh pineapple contains a good amount of vitamin C, bromelain, an enzymatic protein which aids in digestion, respiratory and inflammation, and manganese. Manganese is a trace mineral in the body, responsible for nutrient absorption, bone development and wound healing.

Ingredients:

- 1 Cup of Pineapple
- ½ Cup of Orange Juice
- ½ Cup of Pomegranate Juice
- ½ Cup of Milk
- 2 Scoop of Whey Protein Powder
- 3-4 Ice cubes

Directions:

1. Crush ice in blender.
2. Combine all ingredients and blend to desired consistency.

Sweet and tart, strawberries continue to be one of the most popular berries because they are delicious and full of antioxidants! Your taste buds get a full-flavor treatment when you ingest one of these beauties! Naturally low in calories, high in nutrients and minerals, and serve as awesome antioxidants because they have high amounts of phytochemicals and vitamin C. They are also chocked full of the family of B vitamins: niacin, riboflavin, folic and panothenic acid. This high content of B vitamins helps the body metabolize proteins, carbohydrates and fats. So stock up on the ever amazing strawberry!!! It's too good to pass up! Strawberries are now grown year-round, but if you can't find fresh, frozen is good for you, too!

Ingredients:

- 1 Cup of Strawberry
- ½ Cup of Fresh Cream
- ½ Cup of Milk
- 1 Scoop of Strawberry Protein Powder

Directions:

1. Remove green stem and slice strawberries. (If you cannot tolerate the seeds, puree strawberries then strain through a fine strainer or triple-folded cheesecloth.)
2. Combine cream, milk and protein powder into blender. Blend to desired consistency.

Combining fruit and greens in a smoothie packs a ton of nutrients and minerals into your system. The nutritional benefits of combining fruits with greens supercede any other combination in regard to detoxification. It's is recommended to use fresh cherries, however, because they are highly seasonal, frozen cherries work as a great substitute! The chocolate milk provides just enough sweetness to counter the tartness of the cherries.

Ingredients:

- 1 Cup of Cherries
- 1 Cup of Spinach Leaves
- 2 Scoop of Whey Protein Powder
- 1 Cup Chocolate Milk

Directions:

1. Remove stems and rinse cherries.
2. Add remaining ingredients and puree to desired consistency.

The name suggests an interesting combination of berries and greens, however, the avocado is actually the "fruit" of a tree. So, this is basically a fruit-fruit smoothie. Highly nutritious, this smoothie rewards your body with many and various vitamins, minerals, calories and antioxidants. There's no sodium or cholesterol--only potassium (more than a banana!), healthy mono-saturated fats and fiber. Be sure to purchase a high quality, non-alcoholic vanilla extract for optimal flavor and results.

Ingredients:

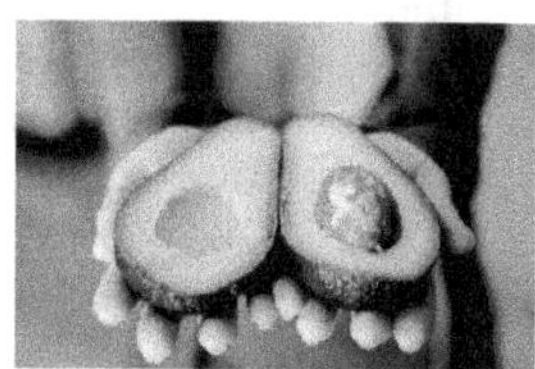

- ¼ Cup milk
- ¾ Cup plain or vanilla yogurt
- 1 Whole banana
- 1 ½ Cup frozen strawberries
- ¼ avocado
- ¼ tsp Vanilla extract

Directions:

1. Slice avocado in half lengthwise. Scoop out pulp and place in blender.
2. Add banana, yogurt and milk to blender. Puree until blended thoroughly.
3. Add strawberries. Puree to desired consistency.
4. While blending, add vanilla extract.

This yogurt-based drink provides an ample amount of antioxidants, protein, potassium, calcium and vitamins C and A to get you through a better part of the day. If yogurt isn't for you, try substituting plain Kefir. Kefir and yogurt are both cultured milks, however, Kefir is more liquid and offers approximately three times the amount of probiotic cultures than yogurt. Another difference is, while yogurt passes through your body, the probiotics in Kefir plant themselves in your digestive tract and attack any "bad bacteria".

Ingredients:

- 3/4 Cup Plain Yogurt
- 5 large frozen Strawberries
- 1 Banana
- 2 Tbsp Peanut Butter
- 2 Tbsp Milk

Directions:

1. Combine banana, yogurt (or Kefir) and milk in a blender. Puree until blended.
2. Add strawberries and peanut butter. Combine to desired consistency.

ELVIS SMOOTHIE

The King loved a simple peanut butter and banana sandwich, and if was good enough for The King, it's good for all! Quick, easy and delicious, there's just no reason to pass this up! The combination provides ample protein, fiber, potassium, magnesium, and probiotics, to keep you satiated for hours. Having a hard time getting vitamins and minerals into the kiddos? Try this once.... you might even sneak a few heart-healthy flax seeds... they'll be begging for more!

Ingredients:

- 3/4 Cup plain or vanilla yogurt
- 2 Tbs Peanut Butter
- 1 Banana
- 1/8 Cup milk
- 3/4 Cup ice

Directions:

1.   Combine all ingredients and blend thoroughly. Puree until desired consistency.

CHOCO-NANA SMOOTHIE

This go-to quick smoothie has chocolate!!! Studies have shown that a moderate amount of dark chocolate is good for you! A high quality dark chocolate (70-85%) provides antioxidants, and a ton of minerals we need, (but don't really think about), including copper, manganese, magnesium and iron. Additional potassium from the banana and probiotics from yogurt provide a healthy, satisfying way to get that chocolate fix! The chocolate blends best if it is room temperature.

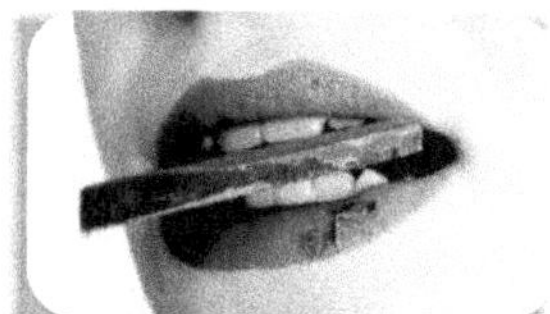

Ingredients:

- ¼ Cup milk
- ¾ Cup plain or vanilla yogurt
- 1 Banana
- 3 Dove Chocolates (dark) or roughly 2-3 Tbsp Chips
- 1 Cup ice

Directions:

1.   Combine all ingredients into blender. Puree to desired consistency.

Whoever thought of combining peanut butter and chocolate was genius! This sweet smoothie packs in less than 600 calories and provides potassium, probiotics and antioxidants. High in protein, it will keep you going through those tough days.

Ingredients:

- ¼ Cup milk
- ¾ Cup plain or vanilla yogurt
- 1 Banana
- 2-3 Tbsp Dark Chocolate Chips
- 1 Cup ice
- 2 Tbsp Peanut Butter

Directions:

1. Combine all ingredients until smooth.

PURPLE SMOOTHIE

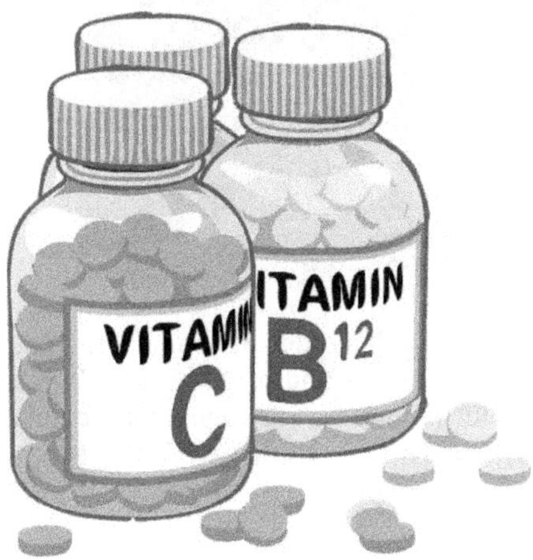

This berry combination makes this smoothie a beautiful purple! Additionally, it's full of vitamins C and A, as well as antioxidants. Potassium comes from the banana and the cinnamon is optional. If you aren't crazy about cinnamon, you might try a sprinkle of nutmeg or pumpkin pie spice.

Ingredients:

- 1/8 Cup milk
- 1/2 Cup plain yogurt
- 1 Whole banana
- 1/2 Cup frozen strawberries
- 1/2 Cup frozen blueberries
- Cinnamon, to taste

Directions:

1. Combine milk, yogurt and banana in blender. Puree until thoroughly combined.
2. Add frozen berries. Puree to desired consistency.
3. Sprinkle lightly with cinnamon, or other spice.

HONEY BUTTER SMOOTHIE

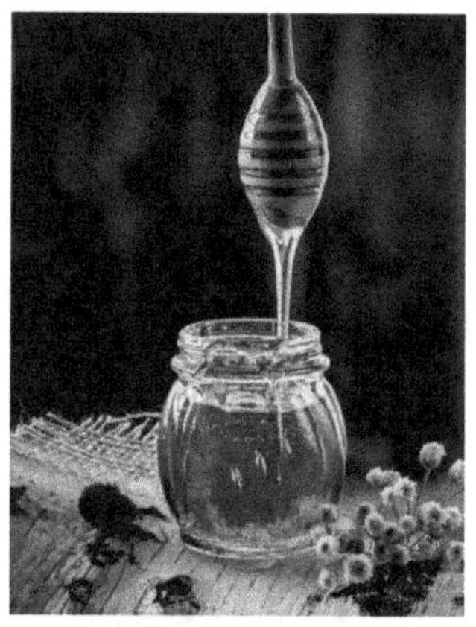

If you like peanut butter with a touch of honey, this smoothie is for you! It provides a variety of nutrients and protein, as well as heart-healthy oils from the nuts. Walnuts, almonds, pine nuts, macadamia nuts, flax seeds, pumpkin and sunflower seeds all work great in this recipe.

Ingredients:

- 1 Cup Milk
- 1 Ripe Banana
- 1/4 Cup Mixed Nuts
- 2 Tbsp Peanut butter
- 2 Scoop Whey protein powder
- 2 Tsp Honey
- 1 Tsp Cocoa powder

Directions:

1. Combine milk, banana and nuts in blender. Puree to desired consistency.
2. Add protein powder. Puree until blended thoroughly.
3. Add cocoa and honey. Blend to desired consistency.

SWEET CINNAMON SMOOTHIE

Cinnamon offers an array of medicinal benefits. It has anti-inflammatory properties, as well as antioxidant properties in the form of polyphenols. It may also contribute to minimizing the risks of cardiac disease, blood pressure and high cholesterol. This sweet smoothie derives its sweetness from maple syrup and vanilla extract, as well as the banana. It is recommended to use alcohol-free vanilla extract and a high quality maple syrup with no added sugar. Nut garnishes might include macadamia nuts, toasted almonds, or pumpkin seeds.

Ingredients:

- 2 medium banana, sliced
- 1 tsp. nutmeg
- 1 tsp. cinnamon
- 1 tsp. vanilla extract
- 1 tsp. maple syrup
- Almond milk to fill line
- Nuts as garnish
- Shredded Coconut as garnish

Directions:

1. Combine all ingredients into blender and puree to desired consistency.
2. Top with garnish (optional)

If you have truly found value in my publication please take a minute and rate my book, I'd be eternally grateful if you left a review. As an independent author I rely on reviews for my livelihood and it gives me great pleasure to see my work is appreciated.

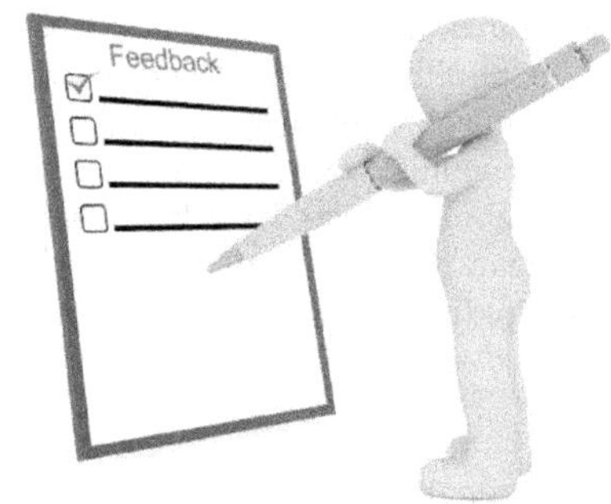

www.ingramcontent.com/pod-product-compliance
Lightning Source LLC
Chambersburg PA
CBHW050807240726
48654CB00008B/666